Alkaline Ketogenic Superfoods

Heal Your Body, Stimulate Massive Weight Loss and Look Amazing (without feeling hungry, bored, or deprived)

By Elena Garcia
Copyright Elena Garcia © 2020

All rights reserved. No part of this publication may be reproduced, stored in a retrieval system, or transmitted, in any form or by any means, electronic, mechanical, photocopying, recording or otherwise, without the prior written permission of the author and the publishers.

The scanning, uploading, and distribution of this book via the Internet or via any other means without the permission of the author are illegal and punishable by law. Please purchase only authorized electronic editions, and do not participate in or encourage electronic piracy of copyrighted materials.

Disclaimer

A physician has not written the information in this book. It is advisable that you visit a qualified dietician so that you can obtain a highly personalized treatment for your case, especially if you want to lose weight effectively. This book is for informational and educational purposes only and is not intended for medical purposes. Please consult your physician before making any drastic changes to your diet.

All information in this book has been carefully researched and checked for factual accuracy. However, the author and publishers make no warranty, expressed or implied, that the information contained herein is appropriate for every individual, situation or purpose, and assume no responsibility for errors or omission. The reader assumes the risk, and full responsibility for all actions and the author will not be held liable for any loss or damage, whether consequential, incidental, and special or otherwise, that may result from the information presented in this publication.

<u>The book is not intended to provide medical advice or to take the place of medical advice and treatment from your personal physician.</u> Readers are advised to consult their own doctors or other qualified health professionals regarding the treatment of medical conditions. The author shall not be held liable or responsible for any misunderstanding or misuse of the information contained in this book. <u>The information is not intended to diagnose, treat, or cure any disease.</u> It's merely an inspiration to live a healthy lifestyle. If you suffer from any medical condition, are pregnant, lactating, or on medication, <u>be sure to talk to your doctor</u> before making any drastic changes in your diet and lifestyle.

When choosing foods for preventing disease and achieving good health, it is important to remember that the overall diet and eating patterns are the most important factors. It is better to eat a diet rich in a variety of nutrient-dense foods than to concentrate on individual foods.

Be sure to talk to a qualified dietician before making any drastic changes to your diet.

Table of Contents

Introduction 10
The Alkaline Keto Lifestyle Explained 15
The Keto Super Powerful Basics 15
Alkaline Diet - Powerful Detox & Alkaline Minerals to Help You Feel Amazing 19
    The Common Mistakes with the Ketogenic Diet (Can Make You Sick and Prevent Healthy Weight Loss) 23
    The Life-Changing Role of Alkaline Foods 24
What Do Alkaline and Keto Diets Have in Common? 26
Watercress – Your Natural Hydration Spa 28
Watercress Recipes 33
    Green Fat Burner Smoothie 33
    Massive Green Energy Watercress Smoothie 34
    Easy Watercress Nuts Salad 35
Cucumber – The Optimal Alkaline Hydration & Holistic Beauty Spa 36
    Smoked Salmon Cucumber Salad 40
Easy Hydrating Alkaline Juice 41
    Tasty Mediterranean Olive Bowl 42
Not Strictly Keto 3 Ingredient Salad 43
Beets – Beautiful Color & Beautiful Nutrients 44
Beetroot Recipes 47
    Veggie Lover Juice with Beets 47
    Alkalizing Beetroot Smoothie Soup 48
    Colorful Soulful Salad 49
Avocado – The Miraculous Fatty Fruit 50
Avocado Recipes 54
    Healing Creamy Smoothie 54

- Immune System Boosting Avocado Smoothie 55
- Nutritious Raw Soup Bowl 56

Arugula – Leafy Greens That Actually Taste Good? 57

Arugula Recipes 59
- Simple Arugula Green Keto Smoothie 59
- Green Mineral Balance Smoothie 60
- Arugula Tuna with Lemon Parsley Dressing 61
- Green Veggie Salad with Olives 62
- The Shot of Green Health 63

Almonds – Crunchy & Nutritious Guilt-Free Snack 64

Almond Recipes 68
- Super Low Carb Bowl 68
- Bullet Proof Creamy Coffee Bowl 69
- Almond Ginger Soup 70
- How to Make Almond Milk 71

Asparagus – A Humble Green Superfood 72

Asparagus Recipes 75
- Tasty Low Carb Breakfast 75
- Veggies in a Cave 77
- Creamy Asparagus Soup 78

Tomato – The Common-Sense Superfood 79

Healthy Alkaline Keto Recipes with Tomatoes 81
- The Healthy Skin Glow Bowl 81
- Tomato Alfalfa Soup 82
- Fresh Tomato Gazpacho 83
- Tomato Cilantro Relish 84

Celery – The Simple Everyday Superfood 85

Recipes with Celery 87

- Celery Juice for Energy & Weight Loss 87
- On the Go Celery Juice Shot (Liver Lover) 88
- Easy Energy Reboot Juice..89
- Crazy Keto No Sugar Smoothie..90
- Cucumber Kale Alkaline Keto Smoothie 91

Fennel – The Bulb of Vitality..92
- How to Add More Fennel to Your Diet 94
- Energy Fennel Juice 95
- Sweet Balance Juice 96
- Fennel Salad Dressing...97
- Fennel Detox Soup 97
- Grapefruit –Why Is It Healthier Than Orange?....................................98
- Hormone Rebalancer Natural Energy Smoothie...............................102
- Grapefruit Fat Burner Smoothie 103
- Delicious Vitamin C Power House 104
- Grapefruit Weight Loss Tonic..105

Coconut Oil Magic – The All In One Solution?.......................................106
Coconut Oil Recipes..111
Green Dream Weight Loss Smoothie 111
- Immune System Energy Smoothie...112
- Coconut Oil Cortado Style Coffee Recipe 113
- Creamy Cinnamon Latte Recipe 114
- Green Tea Weight Loss Drink 115
- Easy Creamy Warm Salmon Salad 116
- Ridiculously Easy Sweet Alkaline Keto Balls.....................................117

Introduction

Hello, my Beautiful Health Freaks! Welcome to the next book in the Alkaline Keto Diet series. I created this book to show you that living a healthy lifestyle doesn't have to be hard or complicated.

In fact, it can be as simple as learning about a few superfoods so that you can supercharge your health and wellbeing without having to follow any restrictive diets.

Another benefit is that all the superfoods covered in this book are easy to find. No, this is not another book about spirulina or some green powders you have never even heard of.

(I have nothing against green powders by the way, but, in this book, we will take a different approach, an approach that is both practical and natural).

Vibrant health is all about *Your Inner Resourcefulness*. My number one goal is to empower you. I want to show you that it's not about some complicated health rituals or expensive supplements from overseas. True empowerment comes from a deeper understanding of the simplest (and the most effective) superfoods, such as alkaline keto superfoods!

It's mind-blowing to discover how a few simple diet and lifestyle tweaks can radically transform your health and life! And this book will teach you how you can make those "healthy tweaks" with alkaline ketogenic superfoods.

Alkaline Keto Superfoods - Introduction

But before we get into it, let's make sure we are on the same page. The word "alkaline" is being thrown around in many health communities, and I have noticed that some people believe it's some kind of an overnight cure. Some people think it's about some "spiritual vibration" of foods. Some automatically associate "alkaline" with an immediate remedy to everything. At the same time, many people worship yet another alkaline guru believing everything they say, without actually understanding what alkaline foods and alkaline-inspired diets are all about. Then, there is also the "keto" part, another diet that some people may call a fad...

So, what exactly are alkaline ketogenic superfoods? Some pseudoscientific, complicated ketosis-stimulating or pH-alternating substances? Some new online health fads? The latest nutritional religion? Who knows what!

Well, I am a very practical lady, and as such, I always say - it doesn't have to be complicated. To keep it simple, alkaline keto foods are healthy, natural foods that are good for you and for your health. *(whether you follow an alkaline diet, or a keto diet, or both, or whether you follow something else, you can always benefit from enriching your diet with some good, healthy fats!).* What makes them so amazing is that they are very rich in nutrients and alkaline minerals. At the same time, they are free of gluten, wheat, and other nasty stuff, that, as a health-conscious person you already know are not good for you.

So, here's precisely what you will discover in this simple, practical, no-fluff guide:

1. The basics of the alkaline and keto diets (and why it's not about changing your pH.) You will also discover how you can

Alkaline Keto Superfoods - Introduction

benefit from both diets, even without being 100% perfect. In other words, you will find a few simple, yet powerful diet tweaks that will help you live a healthier lifestyle, have more energy, and, if desired, lose weight. Many people have also been able to heal their bodies and get rid of pain, inflammation, or even diabetes, just by following a more alkaline-keto friendly diet.

(This book is not aimed at diagnosing or curing any specific health conditions; for that, you need to be talking to your doctor/ medical health professional first. This is a simple wellness recipe book inspired by alkaline and keto diets to give you ideas and inspiration.

I want to empower you and offer you the information and motivation you need to live a healthier lifestyle; however, please note, none of my books is designed as a cure, remedy or program for serious health problems).

2. Then, I will briefly introduce you to a few powerful alkaline keto lifestyle tweaks so that you can create balance, enjoy more energy and vitality, and feel amazing!

3. You will also learn what all alkaline keto superfoods have in common and how to incorporate more of them into your diet for better health!

Finally, we will focus on the main characters of this booklet – *Alkaline Ketogenic Superfoods!* Each section of this book will be focusing on a different superfood, what it's known for, and, most importantly, how to add more of it to your diet) through delicious and nutritious recipes you will fall in love with! All of the recipes are simple-to-follow and don't require hours in the kitchen. How cool is that?

It's all about practical and straightforward recipes you can start experimenting with and benefiting from, even before you are done with reading this book!

So, without any further ado, let's get down to it!

Alkaline Keto Superfoods - Introduction

This is the 9th book in the Alkaline Keto series. The series includes:

Book 1: *Alkaline Ketogenic Mix*

Book 2: *Alkaline Ketogenic Smoothies*

Book 3: *Alkaline Ketogenic Juicing*

Book 4: *Alkaline Ketogenic Salads*

Book 5: *Alkaline Ketogenic Green Smoothies*

Book 6: *Alkaline Ketogenic Lifestyle for Massive Weight Loss*

Book 7: *Low Carb Low Sugar Smoothie Bowls*

Book 8: *Alkaline Ketogenic Oils*

You will find them on Amazon & our Website:

www.yourwellnessbooks.com/books

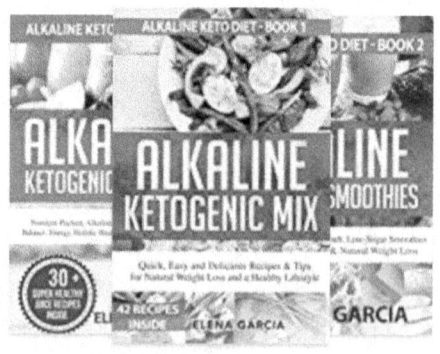

The Alkaline Keto Lifestyle Explained

So, what exactly is the alkaline keto diet and lifestyle?

The simplest definition of the alkaline keto lifestyle is:
it's a brilliant hybrid diet that focuses on the nourishing, mineral-rich power of alkaline foods and the fat-burning power of keto foods.

To understand how this powerful combo works, let's have a quick look at each diet.

The Keto Super Powerful Basics

To make it as simple as possible, the ketogenic diet is a diet low in carbs and high in healthy fats (and moderate in protein).

It's about reducing the carbs while adding in good, healthy fats (more on healthy vs. unhealthy fats later). This cutback in carbs puts your body into a metabolic state called ketosis.

When in ketosis, your body becomes super-efficient at burning fat for energy. A ketogenic diet can also help reduce blood sugar and insulin levels.

Transition your diet into a more keto-friendly diet. It means fewer sugars and carbs and more good fats while eating well!

Following this simple rule (even without going keto full-time) will help you transform your health and feel more energized.

The benefits of the ketogenic diet:

-it manages your sugar levels, prevents diabetes

-it normalizes your hormones and auto-immune system

-it's great for neurological health

Also, your brain will thrive. While it can use both glucose and fats for fuel, ketones are a really clean energy source. I can now concentrate much better and for much longer, while feeling less tired.

Here are other benefits of aligning your dietary choices with a ketogenic-friendly way:

-you will experience reduced hunger and reduced cravings

-you will be burning fat and reducing carbs and so normalizing your insulin levels

-you will protect your heart while raising the good cholesterol

-you will enjoy the anti-age benefits, as keto foods promote longevity and vitality (while nobody ever promised us we would live forever, by deciding to stay healthy, we make sure that the time we are here on earth, we feel good and are vibrant).

In other words- burning crappy carbs for energy is like burning dirty fuel. However, burning fat is a much cleaner fuel while avoiding brain fog. Your brain thrives on ketones.

So, here's what the ketogenic diet consists of:

-75%- 80% fat (don't worry, it's all good fat and will not make you fat).

-5-15% healthy, clean protein

-5% good, unprocessed carbs (yea, you can still eat some carbs and the carbs we will be focusing on, will be healthy unprocessed, no sugar carbs, so no worries, there is no starvation involved here).

The good news is that you can benefit from keto, even without doing it full-time. So many of my readers and friends have been telling me: "It all sounds great, but I don't think I could follow this diet all the time".

Well, the number one tip I can give you is – start making gradual changes. It's as simple as:

-reducing sugars and carbs

-adding more good fats into your diet

Oils to avoid:

-industrial seed oil, trans-fatty acid

- industrial vegetable oils- they are very processed, very corrosive to our arteries, they produce heart disease

-Soybean oil

-Sunflower oil

-Cottonseed oil

-Corn oil

-Canola oil (rapeseed oil)

Condiments like mayonnaise also contain the above-mentioned toxic oils, and so do industrially made bakes and goods.

The fast-food industry uses those oils too.

Instead, you want to focus on healthy, alkaline ketogenic oils, such as:

-coconut oil

-olive oil

-avocado oil

-flaxseed oil

-sesame oil

-grass-fed butter or ghee

Personally, my favorite oils are coconut oil (for cooking and healthy keto fat bombs or no-cook desserts), olive oil (for salads, for veggie smoothies, or certain types of traditional Mediterranean cuisine), and avocado oil (also for salads and all kinds of smoothies).

Alkaline Diet - Powerful Detox & Alkaline Minerals to Help You Feel Amazing

One of the health benefits of alkaline foods and lifestyle is detoxification. First, you are going to be cutting out processed foods that are continually adding toxins to your system (such as wheat, sugar, gluten, nasty chemicals etc.)

Secondly, you are going to be eating foods that allow your body to detox and rid itself of the acids that have built up in your system all this time. We are talking – nutrient and mineral dense alkaline superfoods!

When we detoxify our bodies, we can operate at our optimal levels.

So...what about the pH? All alkaline books talk about it, right?

Our bodies function optimally when our blood is at about 7.365 - 7.45 pH. Now, here's one thing to understand (so many people get this wrong!).

The alkaline <u>diet is not about changing or "raising" your pH</u>. This is where many alkaline guides and gurus can be a bit misleading. You see, our body is smart enough to **self-regulate** our pH for us, no matter what we eat.

Ok, so does it make any sense even to try and eat those alkaline veggies and greens? If we can't change our pH and our body regulates everything for us, what's the point?

Unfortunately, when you constantly bombard your body with acid-forming foods (for example, processed foods, fast food, alcohol, sugar, and even too much meat) you torture your body with incredible stress. Why? Well, because it has to work harder to maintain that optimal pH...

Here's a very simple example...

Imagine you immerse yourself in a bath filled with ice. You say, but hey, my body can self-regulate its optimal temperature, right? And yes, it can. But it will eventually collapse, and you will get ill. The same happens with nutrition and the blood's pH.

You can spend years indulging in toxic, processed, acid-forming foods that only deprive your body of its vital nutrients, saying: "But hey, my body will self-regulate its optimal blood pH."

And again, it will...but sooner or later, it will give up and manifest a disease. It will accumulate fat as its natural defense function to protect your body from over-acidity. We don't wanna end up there, right?

So, to sum up- the alkaline diet is a natural, holistic system, a nutritional lifestyle that advocates the consumption of fresh, unprocessed foods that are rich in alkaline nutrients. These are called alkaline foods, and they help your body stimulate its optimal healing functions. Yes! A healthy body needs nutrients, and fresh low sugar fruits and vegetables are great for that.

Shifting your diet to one that is full of alkaline foods is one of the easiest and best things you can do for your overall health. And the best thing is- we will be combining alkaline foods with keto-friendly meals to make it easy, delicious and fun! Much simpler to follow for the long term.

What I like about the alkaline diet is that you don't have to be 100% perfect. It's enough to make sure you add a ton of greens and veggies and make your diet rich in alkaline foods. With this book, you can get started right away! You will know the best alkaline superfoods that are inexpensive and easy to find in your local supermarket. And, the recipes will teach you how to incorporate these foods into your diet, using delicious salads, smoothies, healing elixirs, and other amazing food combinations.

Another thing worth mentioning is that when it comes to the alkaline diet, there is something called the 70/30 rule meaning that about 70% of your diet should be fresh, nutrient-dense alkaline-forming foods and the remaining 30% can be acid-forming foods (however they still should be clean and organic, for example, grass-fed meat or organic eggs).This is what a hybrid alkaline keto lifestyle is all about. Healthy greens, vegetables, quality animal products, and good fats.

Simple. Balanced. Flexible. Common-sense!

Nothing is too strict. It's not about going hungry or reducing your calories. If anything, you want to eat more! More of nutrient-rich alkaline and keto foods.

The better you feel, and the more weight you lose (if weight loss is your goal) , the more addictive this lifestyle gets! Of course, we are talking about good addiction here.

Alkaline Keto Basics – the Holistic Approach to Health

While this book focuses on the most nutritious and essential alkaline keto foods, we have also created a full printable alkaline keto food lists to help you on your journey. To get our recommended alkaline keto food lists, visit our private website at:

www.yourwellnessbooks.com/alkalineketo

The alkaline keto food lists will help you identify which foods you should be eating more of so that you can feel confident knowing you are getting closer to your wellness and weight loss goals.

(any problems with your download, please email: info@yourwellnessbooks.com)

The Common Mistakes with the Ketogenic Diet (Can Make You Sick and Prevent Healthy Weight Loss)

The most common mistake that people make is that they do not include enough veggies and greens with their keto foods. That can cause imbalance and acidity. Hence, I am such a big fan of keto and alkaline diets combined. Green vegetables are a fantastic addition to your keto diet.

They will help you have more energy and also add more variety to your diet.

The real keto lifestyle is about variety, abundance, and energy. It's hard to be successful with a keto diet if a menu consists entirely of animal products.

Many people avoid all fruit on the keto diet. And, there is certainly a reason behind it. Most fruits are rich in carbs and sugars. However, there are many fruits you can enjoy. We are talking about low-sugar and high nutrient alkaline keto fruits, such as:

-avocados

-limes

-lemons

-grapefruit

-tomatoes

Yes, even though acidic in taste, limes, lemons, and grapefruits are actually alkaline to the body. The reason for that is that they are very low in sugar and high in nutrients as well as alkaline minerals. The taste can sometimes be misleading!

The Life-Changing Role of Alkaline Foods

It's important to get a ton of greens, and alkaline foods as these foods are rich in minerals and vitamins while at the same time don't contain sugar.

I have been promoting alkaline foods for years.

They oxygenate your body and help you have more energy and can be combined with other diets such as paleo or keto diet.

In its optimal design, alkaline diet advocates using quality plant-based oils such as avocado and olive oil, and coconut oil, and it also excludes wheat products and crappy carbs.

Foods that are rich in sugar are also excluded. As already mentioned, the alkaline diet includes low sugar fruits (limes, lemons, grapefruits, etc.)

One of the main principles of the alkaline diet is adding a ton of green veggies into your diet.

The best way to be adding these alkaline foods is via veggie smoothies and juices. The recipe section of this book will give you some ideas. There are also many fantastic alkaline-friendly drinks that will not only help you re-energize and alkalize your body without messing around with your keto lifestyle but will also bring more variety into your diet. Many of these drinks will help you feel more relaxed and balanced.

They will also help you quit drinking sugary drinks, and harmful, chemical-packed sodas and, in many cases, can also help you reduce your caffeine intake. It's a great feeling if you can just wake up and go without depending on caffeine and sugar and feeling moody all the time. Of course, if you enjoy the taste of coffee- go for it. Everything is OK in moderation. However, the best thing you can do, both for your body and mind, is to get energy naturally, from alkaline keto superfoods!

So, let the journey begin!

In case you haven't done so already, be sure to get your printable alkaline keto food lists for extra study:

www.yourwellnessbooks.com/alkalineketo

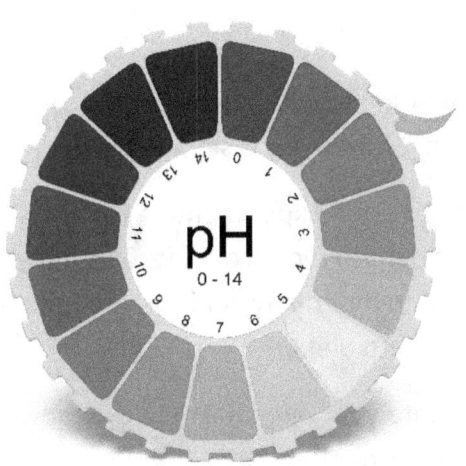

What Do Alkaline and Keto Diets Have in Common?

Even though at first sight, alkaline and keto diets may seem to be very different, there are also many similarities. For example:

-both diets stay away from all forms of sugar, even fructose (hence both alkaline and keto diets focus on low sugar fruit).

-both diets stay away from processed carbs, gluten, and wheat

-both diets like leafy greens and veggies

-both diets like good fats and healthy oils

Also, alkaline diet is not the same as vegan (it can be, but it doesn't have to). There are many "alkalarians" who also consume some quality animal products (such as fresh-caught fish, or grass-fed meat, butter etc.) with their veggies.

At the same time, the keto diet doesn't have to be about going hardcore "carnivore." Nothing is set in stone.

It's all about learning and experimenting for yourself and choosing what you think is right for you, your lifestyle and your body. The bottom line is – there are many kinds of alkaline diets, and there are many kinds of keto diets.

You can easily create your own diet, just by following a few simple guidelines from this book!

So, without further ado, let's learn more about the best alkaline keto superfoods you can start adding to your diet without breaking the bank!

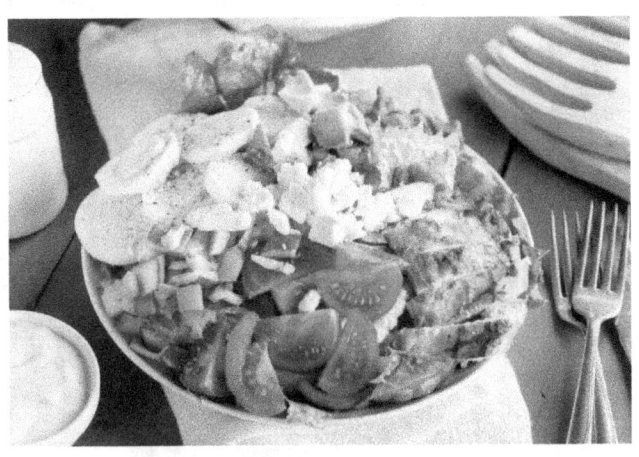

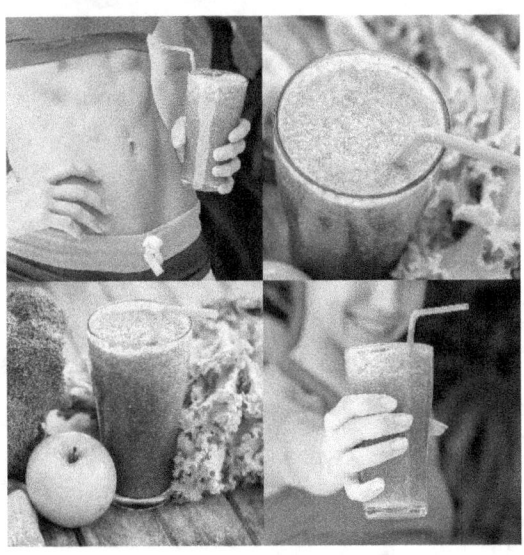

Watercress – The Tasty Green

While everyone is looking for the latest green powder fad, the most hydrating and nutritious greens such as watercress, are very often overlooked.

With its original, peppery, slightly spicy taste (similar to mustard and wasabi), watercress can be a fantastic addition to your salads, veggie smoothies, or gluten-free wraps.

The best part? Like all (or most) superfoods covered in this book, it is easy to find in your local supermarket and grocery store. It's also full of health benefits, such as:

1. **It's Very Rich in Vitamin K as Well as Other Nutrients.**

Watercress is amazing natural weight-loss food as it is very low in calories and super high in nutrients (hence it's been labeled as an extremely nutrient-dense food).

It's especially rich in Vitamin K, which is a fat-soluble vitamin we need for healthy bones and blood clotting.

As far as its main nutrients go, one cup of watercress (about 34 grams), consists of:

Calories: 4

Carbs: 0.4 grams

Protein: 0.8 grams

Fat: 0 grams

Fiber: 0.2 grams

Vitamin A: 22% of the Reference Daily Intake (RDI)

Vitamin C: 24% of the RDI

Vitamin K: 106% of the RDI

Calcium: 4% of the RDI

Manganese: 4% of the RDI

So, if you are concerned with your bone health, try adding more watercress to your diet. Even 1 cup of watercress added to your salads or smoothies can do true wonders to your body.

2. It's Very Rich in Natural Antioxidants

Watercress contains a lot of natural compounds called antioxidants. These are designed as natural protection against cell damage caused by free radicals (these can provoke oxidative stress and lead to over-acidity in the body)

By eating a diet rich in antioxidant-rich foods you prevent the risk of oxidative stress while protecting yourself from many preventable diseases.

Watercress is one of the most alkaline and nutritious leafy greens you could ever get (and it tastes better than kale and spinach).

3. Great for Optimal Heart Health & Reduced Inflammation

As a cruciferous vegetable, watercress is very beneficial for optimal heart health.

It's very abundant in antioxidants such as beta carotene, zeaxanthin, and lutein. Low levels of these carotenoids are very often linked to heart disease and high blood pressure.

Watercress is also rich in dietary nitrates. Nitrates' main job is to boost blood vessel health by reducing inflammation and decreasing the stiffness of the blood vessels. At the same time, it may also contribute to lower cholesterol levels.

4. Natural Alkaline Protection Against Osteoporosis

Watercress is very rich in natural alkaline minerals such as calcium, magnesium, potassium, and phosphorus. These are very beneficial for optimal bone health. What makes it the real game-changer, though, it's the above-mentioned high level of the Vitamin K content.

Yes, Calcium in itself is already great for bone health. But, combined, vitamin K and potassium, it can be more effective.

This is why a balanced, healthy diet that is rich in nutrient-dense vegetables is associated with natural bone health.

5. Promotes a Super Healthy Immune System

Watercress is pretty rich in Vitamin C. In fact, 1 cup of watercress covers about 20% of the recommended daily intake of this precious Vitamin.

Vitamin C is essential for a healthy immune system, and its deficiency has been linked to increased inflammation as well as decreased immune ability.

You need Vitamin C to increase the production of white blood cells so that you can fight and even prevent infections more easily.

When it comes to Vitamin C, most people think that the only way to get it naturally is by eating a ton of fruit. And yes, fruit can be good for you in moderation. However, the main problem behind most fruits is their rich sugar content.

I find it very amazing that greens, such as watercress, can also help us boost our Vitamin C intake without adding more sugar or carbs.

6. Amazing Natural Weight Loss Tool

Since watercress is an incredibly nutrient-dense food and is low in calories, it's a fantastic, nutritious, alkaline, and keto-friendly superfood to help you lose weight. Your body might be craving fast food and processed foods, simply because it's deprived of many nutrients. So, if your goal is healthy and sustainable weight loss, start adding more greens such as watercress into your diet.

Aside from being rich in nutrients and high in calories, watercress is also very rich in nitrates. These are natural compounds found in healthy foods such as beets, radishes, and leafy greens (including watercress).

Nitrates relax your blood vessels while increasing the amount of nitric oxide in your blood, hence optimizing exercise tolerance and high performance. This is why so many athletes use leafy greens and superfoods such as watercress. It can be an excellent exercise optimizer (and it's also very hydrating).

7. Contains Natural Carotenoids for a Healthy Eyesight

Watercress is rich in natural antioxidant compounds such as lutein and zeaxanthin, which are essential for natural eye health (lower risk of cataracts and age-related degeneration). This benefit is amplified thanks to the rich content of Vitamin C.

So, How to Add More Watercress to Your Diet?

-Serve it as a side dish with some eggs, fish or meat.

-Use it as a quick snack, with some olive oil, Himalayan salt, avocado, lemon juice and spices

-Add it to your salads and soups (at the end of cooking)

-Add it your sandwiches or gluten-free wraps

-Use it to make a pesto-like sauce (just blend it with some garlic, spices and olive oil)

-Add it to your smoothies and juices

Watercress Recipes

Green Fat Burner Smoothie

This recipe combines the best fat-burning ingredients ever, helps you concentrate for long hours while feeling lighter.

It's also great if you suffer from water retention. I love drinking this smoothie in the summer.

Servings: 2

Ingredients:

- 1 green tea teabag (or 1 teaspoon green tea powder)
- 1 cup of coconut water
- 1 cup water
- 1 big avocado
- 1 big grapefruit
- Half cup watercress
- 1 teaspoon cinnamon powder
- Stevia to sweeten, if needed

Instructions:

1. Boil 1 cup of water.
2. Add in the green tea.
3. Cover.
4. In the meantime, process the remaining ingredients in a blender.
5. Add in the cooled herbal infusion and process again.
6. If needed, sweeten with stevia.
7. Serve chilled and enjoy!

Watercress

Massive Green Energy Watercress Smoothie

If you don't like spinach or kale, I highly recommend you try watercress instead. It's delicious, both in salads and smoothies.

This smoothie is low carb, high fat, alkaline and keto-friendly, and super high in nutrients. All you need to look and feel amazing!

Servings: 2

Ingredients:

- 1 cup watercress leaves, washed
- 1 small avocado, peeled, pitted and sliced
- 4 tablespoons fresh lemon juice
- 1 tablespoon coconut oil
- 2 cups coconut or almond milk, unsweetened
- Himalaya salt and black pepper to taste

Instructions:

1. Place all the ingredients in a blender.
2. Process well until smooth.
3. Serve and enjoy!

Watercress

Easy Watercress Nuts Salad

This simple alkaline keto salad is super delicious and nutritious. It can also be served as a simple side dish to help you add more greens to your diet.

Serves:2
Ingredients
For the Salad:
- A handful of fresh blueberries
- 1 cup of fresh watercress
- 4 tablespoons of chopped walnuts
- 1 big avocado, peeled, pitted and sliced
- A few sardines, or a few slices of smoked salmon

Dressing:
- 1 tablespoon of coconut vinegar (you can also use lime or lemon juice)
- 4 tablespoons of melted coconut oil
- 1/2 teaspoon of low carb mustard
- Some pepper and Himalayan salt to taste

Instructions:
1. Whisk the coconut oil, Dijon mustard, coconut vinegar, ground black pepper, and sea salt in a bowl until the dressing becomes smooth, and you get a well-combined dressing.
2. Combine the watercress with walnuts, strawberries, and avocado and drizzle the prepared dressing over the salad.
3. Toss the salad lightly to mix well and serve immediately. Enjoy!

Cucumber – The Optimal Alkaline Hydration & Holistic Beauty Spa

Cucumbers are very high in vital nutrients and minerals. They are also very hydrating and commonly used in natural beauty treatments.

Very low in calories while offering great hydration and soluble fiber, cucumbers are great for a healthy and sustainable weight loss. Let's have a look at all-natural health benefits of cucumbers:

1. Very High in Vital Nutrients

Cucumbers are low in calories but high in many vital vitamins and minerals.

A 1 cup of raw, unpeeled, cucumber contains, approximately:

Calories: 45

Total fat: 0 grams

Carbs: 11 grams

Protein: 2 grams

Fiber: 2 grams

Vitamin C: 14% of the RDI

Vitamin K: 62% of the RDI

Magnesium: 10% of the RDI

Potassium: 13% of the RDI

Manganese: 12% of the RDI

Additionally, cucumbers are made up of over 90% water and can be turned into a refreshing, alkaline keto-friendly juice.

If you use organic cucumbers, there is no need to peel them, and so you can maximize their rich nutrient content.

2. Full of Natural Antioxidants

Oxidative stress caused by free radicals is very often associated with a weaker immune system. The best way to protect yourself from free radicals is by adding more antioxidant-rich food to your diet.

Luckily, cucumbers are very rich in antioxidants as they contain flavonoids and tannins (the two groups of compounds that are especially effective at fighting free radicals.)

3. Optimal Hydration & Beautiful Skin

Proper hydration is crucial for temperature regulation and the transportation of waste products and nutrients. While drinking water is excellent, you can take your hydration routine to the next level by adding more cucumbers to your diet. You can even juice them or add them to your smoothies.

People very often obsess about some expensive alkaline water technology. In reality, all you need is quality filtered water (I use simple water jar and filters called Britta) and some quality fruits and veggies that are naturally rich in alkaline minerals – cucumber is one of them.

Also, not everyone enjoys drinking plain water. Well, juicing low sugar superfoods, such as cucumbers, can be a great alternative. Moreover, you can keep the fiber and use it as a natural face mask, or add it to your salads.

4. Natural Weight Loss

I think this one is pretty common sense! Cucumbers are low in calories and high in precious nutrients and vitamins to help you stay energized.

You can quickly turn them into guilt-free snacks.

For example, raw cucumbers with freshly made guacamole (avocado, tomato, and olive oil), or coconut avocado cream (just blend avocados, coconut milk, Himalayan salt, and some spices). So easy and yummy and perfect for a quick, alkaline, and keto-friendly snack that is guilt-free.

5. Great for Low Sugar Diets

Since cucumber is naturally low in sugar, it's great for low sugar diet and any diets aimed at diabetics.

You can make delicious, low sugar smoothies and smoothie bowls using cucumbers. For example, you can blend cucumbers and coconut milk (or some Greek yogurt if you prefer) and add some black pepper and Himalayan salt. Then, you can also add some nuts and seeds if you want. So easy, hydrating, and delicious! You could even enjoy it as a simple, detox smoothie-style soup.

6. Excellent for Bowel Movement

Dehydration and low fiber intake may lead to constipation.

Since cucumbers are very high in water and also contain natural fiber, they are a great natural remedy for a regular bowel movement (of course, like with everything, you don't want to overdo it, especially if you are still new to eating clean foods).

How to Add Cucumbers to Your Diet

You can enjoy cucumbers as a quick snack with some natural nut butter, guacamole, or veggie hummus.

You can also juice them or add them to your smoothies and salads. Cucumbers are also a great takeaway snack (especially when combined with some goat cheese, so yummy!).

Cucumbers work great in fruit infused water recipes (especially when combined with some citric fruits such as oranges, limes, and lemons).

Now, let's have a look at my favorite cucumber recipes to help you shine!

Cucumber

Smoked Salmon Cucumber Salad

This salad is delicious, hydrating, filling, and fun. Horseradish cream spices it up and gives it a unique flavor. This salad is perfect as a takeaway lunch that will keep you full until the late afternoon or early evening. The best part? It's very easy to make!

Serves: 1-2

Ingredients:
- 4 big slices of smoked salmon, cut into smaller pieces
- 1 teaspoon of horseradish cream
- 4 big cucumbers, peeled and sliced
- half cup of coconut yogurt or full-fat Greek yogurt
- 1 cup fresh greens of your choice
- A dash of ground black pepper
- Himalayan salt to taste
- 1 tablespoon olive oil

Instructions:
1. Place all the ingredients in a salad bowl. Stir well.
2. Season with black pepper and Himalayan salt to taste.
3. Enjoy!

Cucumber

Easy Hydrating Alkaline Juice

This recipe is one of my favorite juicing recipes. It's simple, very refreshing, full of alkaline nutrients and great for your skin. It's also rich in Vitamin C and helps boost your immune system.

Serves: 1-2

Ingredients:

- 1 big grapefruit, peeled
- 4 big cucumbers, peeled
- 1-inch ginger, peeled

Instructions:

Juice, enjoy, and shine!

***If you don't have a juicer, you can make this recipe in a smoothie version, by adding some coconut milk, and/or water.

Ingredients:

- 1 cup coconut water (or filtered water)
- 1 cup coconut milk
- 1 big grapefruit, peeled
- 4 big cucumbers, peeled
- 1-inch ginger, peeled

Instructions:

Blend all the ingredients in a blender. Process until smooth and enjoy!

Tasty Mediterranean Olive Bowl

If you like Mediterranean flavors and spices, you will love this recipe. Who said smoothie bowls must be sweet? Also, this one is super nutritious and perfect as a quick lunch recipe (or a delicious side dish).

Serves: 1-2

Ingredients for the Smoothie:
- 1 avocado, peeled and pitted
- 1 cup almond milk, unsweetened
- Half cup organic tomato juice
- 1/4 cup mixed Italian herbs
- 2 cucumbers, peeled and cut into smaller pieces
- A handful of arugula leaves
- Himalayan salt and black pepper to taste

Ingredients for the Toppings:
- A handful of pistachios
- A handful of black olives, pits removed
- A handful of green olives, pits removed
- A few fresh basil leaves

Instructions:
1. Blend all the smoothie ingredients in a blender, until nice and creamy.
2. Pour into a bowl.
3. Mix in the rest of the ingredients by placing them on top.
4. Serve and enjoy!

Cucumber

Not Strictly Keto 3 Ingredient Salad

Even though I am grain-free most of the time (I try to stay away from gluten), sometimes I like to use a bit of quinoa in my recipes. Yes, I know, it's not strictly keto. And it's fine with me! What I like about quinoa is that it's naturally gluten-free and very nutritious. I like to use it for quick salads like this one.

However, if you would like to keep it strictly keto and with no grains, feel free to swap quinoa with some tomato slices.

Serves: 1
Ingredients:
- Half cup cooked quinoa, chilled
- 2 hardboiled eggs, peel removed
- 2-3 cucumbers, peeled and sliced
- Olive oil and Himalayan salt to taste

Instructions:
1. Combine all the ingredients in a salad bowl.
2. Mix well, drizzle over some olive oil and Himalayan salt.
3. Enjoy!

Beets – Beautiful Color & Beautiful Nutrients

Beets (or beetroots) are a popular root vegetable that is jam-packed with many essential vitamins and minerals. It has been used in natural medicine for centuries.

The best part? Beets are naturally sweet and delicious, as well as very easy to add to your diet.

So, let's have a look at what beets are known for:

1. Low Calorie and Nutrient Dense Profile

Just like other superfoods discussed so far, beets are very low in calories and super high in nutrients and vitamins (therefore being a great natural weight loss food).

A half-cup (about 120 grams) of cooked beetroot, contains:

Calories: 44

Protein: 1.7 grams

Fat: 0.2 grams

Fiber: 2 grams

Vitamin C: 6% of the RDI

Folate: 20% of the RDI

Vitamin B6: 3% of the RDI

Magnesium: 6% of the RDI

Potassium: 9% of the RDI

Phosphorous: 4% of the RDI

Manganese: 16% of the RDI

Iron: 4% of the RDI

Beets are particularly high in folate - one of the essential B-vitamins needed to make red and white blood cells in the bone marrow. It also converts carbohydrates into energy (perfect for optimal weight loss!).

2. Great for Healthy Blood Pressure & Optimal Performance

Beets are rich in nitrates, which have a blood pressure-lowering effect. At the same time, nitrates can improve physical performance by improving the efficiency of mitochondria (responsible for producing energy in your cells). Therefore, so many cyclists and athletes love fresh beet juice before their training (nitrate levels peak within 2–3 hours after consuming beet juice).

3. Better Digestion

Beets are a good source of natural dietary fiber, which is recommended for healthy digestion.

In fact, one cup of beetroot contains about 3.5 grams of fiber.

Natural fiber may also help reduce the risk of many chronic diseases such as colon cancer and type 2 diabetes.

5. Natural Brain Booster

Beets contain nitrates that may improve mental function by dilating blood vessels and thus increasing blood flow to the brain.

Beets may even improve blood flow to the frontal lobe of the brain (an area associated with thinking), therefore improving memory and decision making.

6. Natural Weight Loss

Beets are low in calories, rich in nutrients and high in water. At the same time, they are rich in fiber (and even some natural protein), which will make you feel full for hours.

I always say that the healthiest way to lose weight is about eating more nutrient-packed, natural foods (such as beetroot and other superfoods featured in this book). You can never go wrong with that, and weight loss doesn't have to be about going hungry.

How to add more beets to your diet:

-you can enjoy them steamed, cooked or even pickled

-they also taste delicious in juices and salads

-beets blended with some coconut yogurt or Greek yogurt make a fantastic dip or salad dressing

-beetroot leaves are very alkaline-forming to the body, so don't throw them out, you can also use them for your juices and smoothies.

Now, let's have a look at some beetroot recipes!

Beetroot Recipes

Veggie Lover Juice with Beets

Servings: 3
Ingredients:
- 3 beets (with greens), peeled
- 3 large tomatoes, cut into smaller pieces
- 1 red bell pepper, chopped
- 1 large celery stalk, chopped
- A handful of mint leaves
- 2 tablespoons avocado oil

Instructions:
1. Juice all the ingredients.
2. Pour into a big jar, combine with avocado oil, serve in smaller glasses, and enjoy!
3. If needed, season with some Himalayan salt.

Beetroot

Alkalizing Beetroot Smoothie Soup

This smoothie can also be used as a dip to be served with some veggies.

It also makes a great meal replacement if you are pressed for time and are looking for an easy and nutritious meal.

Servings: 1-2

Ingredients:

- 2 beets, cooked
- Half avocado, peeled and sliced
- A handful of arugula leaves
- 1 small garlic clove, peeled and minced
- 4 tablespoons lime juice
- Half cup water, filtered
- 2 tablespoons olive oil
- Himalaya salt and black pepper to taste

Instructions:

1. Place all the ingredients in a blender.
2. Process well until smooth.
3. Serve and enjoy!

Colorful Soulful Salad

Artichokes are highly alkalizing and full of magnesium and potassium.
They're the perfect match for beets and other alkaline keto superfoods!

Serves: 1-2
Ingredients:
- 1 cup of canned artichoke hearts, halved
- 2 beets, cooked (or steamed) and sliced
- A few red onion slices
- ½ cup of coconut yogurt or Greek yogurt
- 2 tablespoons of lime juice
- 2 slices of lime to garnish
- A handful of cashews to garnish
- A handful of cilantro to garnish
- Pinch of Himalayan salt to taste

Instructions:
1. Mix all of the salad ingredients in a large bowl.
2. Stir well while adding the coconut yogurt.
3. Season with Himalayan salt. Garnish with cashews, cilantro, and lime slices. Enjoy!

Avocado – The Miraculous Fatty Fruit

The avocado is a pretty unusual fruit combining the best of alkaline and keto diets. But what makes it so special? Well...most fruits consist primarily of carbs and sugar (hence most fruits are off the keto diets and most weight loss plans). However, avocado is different as it is high in fats (while being low carb and low sugar).

Oh, and it's green and full of alkaline nutrients...hence it's also one of the best fruits you could eat on an alkaline diet (whether you eat fully plant-based or not).

I used to be scared of avocados. Like many other people, I used to think that avocados would make me fat. But, after researching all the benefits of avocados, and incorporating them into my diet, I can honestly tell you I couldn't live without them.

So, let's have a closer look at why avocado is so healthy and good for you:

1. **Incredibly Nutritious**

Avocado is famous for its uniquely high nutrient value. It can be added to many dishes (such as sweet, spicy, and sour) for texture and creaminess. It's also great as a natural face mask!

Avocado

Below are some of its most essential nutrients (in 100 grams of serving, approximately one very small avocado):

Vitamin K: 26% of the daily value (DV)
Folate: 20% of the DV
Vitamin C: 17% of the DV
Potassium: 14% of the DV
Vitamin B5: 14% of the DV
Vitamin B6: 13% of the DV
Vitamin E: 10% of the DV

Other nutrients present in avocado include: manganese, copper, iron, zinc, phosphorous, and vitamins A, B1 (thiamine), B2 (riboflavin) and B3 (niacin).

-160 calories
-2 grams of protein
-15 grams of healthy fats
-9 grams of carbs (7 of those are fiber, so there are only 2 net carbs, which is perfect for low carb diets).

2. Very Rich in Potassium

Potassium is an alkaline mineral that unfortunately, lacks in most people's diets.

Its primary function is maintaining electrical gradients in the body's cells. Avocados are even higher in potassium than bananas (unfortunately bananas are also very high in sugar which doesn't make them very compatible with the alkaline and keto diets, avocados seem to be a much better choice).

Making sure you get enough potassium is necessary to care of your blood pressure, heart, and kidneys.

3. Jam-Packed with Healthy Monounsaturated Fatty Acids

Avocado is one of the fattiest plant foods ever (over 75% of its calories come from fat).

However, the majority of the fat in avocado is a monounsaturated fatty acid called oleic acid.

Oleic acid has been linked to many health benefits, such as reduced inflammation.

4. Avocados Help Nutrient Absorption

When it comes to nutrients, the most important thing is your body's ability to absorb them. Since some nutrients are fat-soluble, they need to be combined with fat for your body to benefit from them.

For example, Vitamins A, D, E, and K, as well as antioxidants like carotenoids, are fat-soluble. Adding avocados to your smoothies and salads can help you increase antioxidant and vitamin absorption.

Another benefit is that avocados will make your smoothies taste very creamy!

5. Rich in Potent Antioxidants

Avocados are also high in antioxidants such as the carotenoids lutein and zeaxanthin. These are incredibly beneficial for healthy eyesight, and they may lower your risk of macular degeneration and cataracts.

6. Even Though Full of Fat, Avocados Are Great for Natural Weight Loss

Even though higher in calories, avocados offer quality calories and an incredible nutritional value, as well as natural fiber. And so, they are great as a satisfying snack to help you stay full and energized for hours. Its high nutrient content can help you eat fewer processed calories, therefore helping you live a healthier lifestyle that leads to sustainable and safe weight loss.

Finally, avocados are very easy to add to your diet and blend well with all kinds of ingredients, from sweet to creamy.

So, how to eat more avocados?
-as a quick snack (half avocado with some Himalayan salt and lemon juice can be very satisfying, you can also add your favorite veggies and spices).
-blend in with your smoothies
-add to your salads
-blend with some tomatoes and garlic to make a delicious guacamole
-use for creamy desserts such as: avocados blended with stevia, coconut oil, cashews, and raw cocoa powder can be a fantastic natural dessert! Yummy, creamy and healthy!

Avocado Recipes

Healing Creamy Smoothie

This simple alkaline keto smoothie is rich in vitamin C, fiber, and alkaline minerals such as potassium. It is also very hydrating and replenishing.

Perfect for a simple, green avocado smoothie.

Serves 1-2

Ingredients

- 1 big cucumber, peeled
- 1 tablespoon coconut oil
- Pinch of Himalayan salt
- 4 tablespoons of raw cashews
- 1 cup yogurt (you can use Greek yogurt, or any plant-based coconut or almond yogurt, just be sure to go for no added sugar)
- 1 avocado, peeled and pitted
- Pinch of black pepper to taste
- A small handful of fresh cilantro leaves

Instructions

1. Place all the ingredients in a blender and process until smooth.
2. If needed, season with Himalayan salt and black pepper.
3. Serve in a smoothie bowl or glass and enjoy!

Avocado

Immune System Boosting Avocado Smoothie

This is a super simple alkaline green smoothie that will help you boost your immune system by enriching your diet with vitamin C and a myriad of alkaline minerals. It's naturally sweet and delicious!

Serves 1-2

Ingredients:

- Half lime, peeled
- 1 cup of coconut or almond milk
- 1 big avocado, peeled and pitted
- 1 teaspoon chia seeds
- 1 tablespoon coconut oil
- 1 teaspoon cinnamon powder
- Stevia to sweeten, if needed

Instructions:

1. Place in a blender.
2. Process until smooth.
3. Serve in a smoothie glass and garnish with a wedge of lime.
4. Enjoy!

Avocado

Nutritious Raw Soup Bowl

This creamy bowl is perfect for a quick brunch or lunch. It offers a myriad of nutrients such as B vitamins and iodine from nori and Omega-3s from chia seeds. Perfect for helping you stay energized and nourished.
It's pretty low-carb, high-fat, and very rich in nutrients. To your health, enjoy!

Serves: 2

Ingredients for the Smoothie:
- 2 nori sheets, soaked in water
- 1 cup coconut milk
- 1 avocado, peeled and pitted
- 1 small cucumber, peeled and cut into smaller pieces
- A handful of watercress leaves
- Himalayan salt and black pepper to taste

More Ingredients for the Toppings:
- A handful of pistachios
- A handful of crushed cashews
- Optional: a few chili flakes, if you like it spicy

Instructions:
1. Blend all the ingredients until smooth. Pour into a bowl.
2. Mix in the rest of the ingredients by placing them on top. Enjoy!

Arugula – Leafy Greens That Actually Taste Good?

Arugula is definitely one of my favorite greens. I just find it so much easier than spinach and kale. It tastes so much better!

It's also known as rucola or salad rocket or Italian cress in some countries.

So, what exactly are its benefits, and what makes it so special?

First of all, this delicious green is very rich in fiber and phytochemicals. At the same time, it's low in sugar, calories, carbohydrates, and fat.

It's especially rich in:

1. Calcium -necessary for bone and tooth health as well as muscle and nerve function.

2. Potassium -an important electrolyte and mineral, essential for heart and nerve function. It's also crucial for muscle contraction. At the same time, it helps to reduce the negative effects of sodium (reducing the risk of high blood pressure).

3. Folate, a B vitamin that supports the production of DNA, crucial for pregnant women.

4. Vitamin C to strengthen your immune system while improving the absorption of iron.

5. Vitamin K, important for blood coagulation. If you require a prescription blood thinner, such as warfarin (Coumadin), discuss your vitamin K intake with your doctor before changing your eating habits.

Arugula

6.Vitamin A -a powerful antioxidant that supports the immune system, healthy kidneys, night vision, and cell growth.

A cup of arugula (about 250 grams) contains:

-0.516 g of protein

-0.132 g of fat

-27.7% of vitamin K

-3.2% of calcium

-2.5% of vitamin C

Arugula also contains some levels of iron, folate, magnesium, potassium, and provitamin A.

So, how to add it to your diet?

-use it as a side salad with a bit of extra virgin olive oil, or avocado oil as well as some Himalayan salt, and spices.

-add to any vegetable (or even fruit) salads

-use it to make green smoothies and juices (much tastier than spinach and kale).

-use it to make fresh pesto by blending it with some basil, pine nuts, olive oil, and organic parmesan cheese

So now, let's have a look at some arugula recipes!

Arugula Recipes

Simple Arugula Green Keto Smoothie

This nutritious green smoothie is perfect if your goal is to have more energy. Healthy fats will help you stay full for hours.

Servings: 1-2

- 1 cup fresh coconut milk, unsweetened
- Half cup water, filtered
- 2-inch turmeric, peeled
- A handful of fresh arugula leaves
- Half avocado, peeled and pitted
- 1 tablespoon coconut oil
- 1 teaspoon maca powder
- Stevia to sweeten (optional)

Instructions:

1. Blend all the ingredients in a blender.
2. Serve and enjoy.
3. This drink is great first thing in the morning. But you can also sip on it during the day to enjoy more energy.

Arugula

Green Mineral Balance Smoothie

This delicious green smoothie is creamy, nutritious, and filling. Perfect for a quick healthy breakfast!

Serves: 1-2

Ingredients:

- 1 cup coconut milk, unsweetened
- 1 big avocado, peeled and pitted
- 1 tablespoon coconut oil
- A handful of arugula leaves
- A bit of stevia to sweeten
- 2 tablespoons blueberries (frozen or fresh)

+ a few lime slices and ice cubes to serve if needed

Instructions:

1. Place all the ingredients in a blender.
2. Process until smooth.
3. Serve and enjoy!
4. This smoothie also tastes delicious when chilled or half-frozen.

Arugula

Arugula Tuna with Lemon Parsley Dressing

This salad offers an incredible mix of clean protein, good fats, and superfood greens. The alkaline keto way!

Serves: 2
Ingredients
For the Salad:
- 1 whole scallion, finely chopped
- 2 cups of fresh arugula leaves
- 1 avocado, peeled, pitted and sliced
- Fresh chopped parsley for topping
- 2 cans of organic tuna in olive oil

For the dressing:
- 4 tablespoons of thick coconut milk
- 4 tablespoons of parsley, chopped
- 2 tablespoons organic lemon juice
- 2 pinches of Himalayan salt (you can always add more if you need to)
- A pinch of black pepper and chili (optional)
- 1 big garlic clove, peeled

Instructions:
1. Combine all the salad ingredients in a big salad bowl and toss well.
2. Mix all the salad dressing ingredients using a small hand blender.
3. Pour the dressing over the salad and stir well.
4. Serve and enjoy!

Arugula

Green Veggie Salad with Olives

This salad is an excellent solution if you are looking for a meal replacing salad, something that will keep you full for many hours. It's a great mix of veggies, protein, and healthy, alkaline-keto fats!

Serves: 2
Ingredients
For the Salad:
- A few tablespoons of green olives
- 1 cucumber, peeled and finely chopped
- A few onion rings
- A handful of fresh arugula leaves
- 1 big garlic clove, peeled
- Half cup black olives, pitted
- A few tomato slices
- A few almonds
- 2 cans of tuna

For dressing:
- 2 tablespoons of Dijon mustard
- 2 tablespoons of olive oil
- A few fresh basil and parsley leaves (optional)
- 1 tablespoon of coconut vinegar
- Black pepper to taste

Arugula

Instructions:
1. Combine all the salad ingredients in a big salad bowl and toss well.
2. Mix all the salad dressing ingredients. You can use a small hand blender, or quickly combine and stir all the ingredients in a small bowl.
3. Pour the dressing over the salad and toss well.
4. Sprinkle over a few mint, parsley, and cilantro leaves.
5. Serve and enjoy!

The Shot of Green Health

Serves: 2

Ingredients:
- 1 cup arugula leaves
- 1 carrot, peeled
- 1 cucumber, peeled
- 1 lime, peeled
- 1 tablespoon olive or avocado oil

Instructions:
Place all the ingredients through a juicer.
Juice, pour into a juice glass, and enjoy!

***If you don't have a juicer, you can blend the ingredients with 1 cup of water and 1 cup of coconut water or coconut milk.
You could also use organic tomato juice, black pepper, and Himalayan salt.

Almonds – Crunchy & Nutritious Guilt-Free Snack

People always ask me about healthy snacks on the alkaline keto lifestyle. The answer? Almonds!

They are incredibly nutritious and very abundant in healthy fats, antioxidants, vitamins, and minerals. Their health and wellness benefits are numerous:

1. Rich in Nutrients

Almonds have an amazing nutrient profile.

A handful of almonds (1-ounce, or 28-gram) contains:

Fiber: 3.5 grams

Protein: 6 grams

Fat: 14 grams (9 of which are monounsaturated)

Vitamin E: 37% of the RDI

Manganese: 32% of the RDI

Magnesium: 20% of the RDI

They also contain some copper, vitamin B2 (riboflavin) as well as phosphorus.

Also, a handful of almonds is 161 calories and only 2.5 grams of digestible carbohydrates.

However, it's also worth mentioning that almonds contain phytic acid, which slightly reduces the absorption of some nutrients, such as iron, zinc, and calcium. Still, this shouldn't be a problem with a healthy and balanced diet.

2. Rich in Antioxidants

Antioxidants present in almonds help protect against oxidative stress, preventing molecule damage in your cells while helping reduce inflammation, aging, and many other diseases.

Most of these antioxidants are present in the brown layer of the almond skin; this is why blanched almonds are considered less therapeutic.

3. Very High in Vitamin E

Almonds are very rich in a fat-soluble antioxidant; Vitamin E.

These antioxidants protect your cells from oxidative damage. In fact, 1 ounce of almonds provides about 37% of the recommended daily intake of Vitamin E, making almonds one of the best food sources of this Vitamin.

3.Can Help Control Blood Sugar

Almonds are low in carbs and high in good fats, natural protein, and fiber. This makes them a great food choice for people with diabetes.

It's also rich in Magnesium, which, according to some studies, could also help prevent metabolic syndrome and type 2 diabetes.

4. Blood Pressure Level Control

Low magnesium levels have also been linked to high blood pressure. Magnesium-rich foods such as almonds could add to high blood pressure prevention and control.

5. Cholesterol Levels Control

Snacking on a couple of handfuls of almonds per day could also lead to mild reductions in "bad" LDL cholesterol, potentially reducing the risk of many diseases.

6. Reduced Hunger and Sugar Cravings as well as Natural Weight Loss

Natural protein and healthy fiber present in almonds can quickly help make you feel fuller; therefore, helping you eat less processed calories coming from unhealthy foods. They are just a perfect addition to your morning smoothies and will make you stay full for hours. Almonds also work great as a natural snack to help you stay away from sugars and carbs (that make us all fat, sick, and tired).

How to Add Almonds to Your Diet

-make a natural paleo-style porridge – combine a handful of soaked almonds with a few slices of almonds and coconut milk, you can also add some chia seeds and some other nuts

-add them to your smoothies and smoothie bowls

-blend them into almond nut butter (so yummy and healthy!)

Almonds

-sprinkle some crushed almonds over your salads, soups and other dishes

-enjoy them as a quick, nutritious snack at work or in between meals

-blend with water to make natural almond milk (more in the recipe section).

Almond Recipes

Super Low Carb Bowl

This is a simple superfood smoothie that will help you boost your immune system by enriching your diet with vitamin C and a myriad of alkaline minerals.

Serves 1-2

Ingredients for the Smoothie:
- 1 big lime, peeled
- 1 cup of coconut or almond milk
- A handful of watercress, washed
- 1 tablespoon coconut oil
- 1 teaspoon cinnamon powder
- Stevia to sweeten, if needed

Ingredients for the Toppings:
- 2 tablespoons chia seeds
- 2 tablespoons crushed almonds

Instructions:
1. Place in a blender.
2. Process until smooth.
3. Pour into a bowl, add in the toppings and serve.
4. Enjoy!

Almonds

Bullet Proof Creamy Coffee Bowl

This smoothie is perfect early in the morning to help you concentrate better at work. It combines the antioxidant properties of blueberries with good fats and a bit of coffee. It's creamy, nutritious, and delicious.

Servings: 2
Ingredients for the Smoothie:
- 1 strong expresso (use organic, quality coffee)
- 1 cup almond milk
- Half avocado, peeled and pitted
- 2 tablespoons almonds
- 2 tablespoons coconut oil
- Stevia to sweeten if needed

Ingredients for the Toppings:
- A handful of blueberries
- A few mint leaves
- Half teaspoon cinnamon powder

Instructions:
1. Blend all the ingredients in a blender until smooth.
2. Pour your smoothie into a bowl.
3. Add in the toppings, serve and enjoy!

Almond Ginger Soup

Ginger is alkaline, anti-inflammatory, anti-bacterial, and it will make your soups taste spicy and delicious! It blends well with almonds and other ingredients.

Servings: 2
Ingredients:
- A handful of almonds, soaked in water for at least a few hours
- 1 cup almond milk
- 2 tablespoons coconut oil
- 2-inch ginger, peeled
- Half garlic clove
- 1 big cucumber, peeled
- Pinch of Himalaya salt and black pepper
- 2 lime slices, peeled
- A few avocado slices

Instructions:
1. Blend all the ingredients in a blender.
2. Serve in a soup bowl.
3. Enjoy!

Almonds

How to Make Almond Milk

Serves: 4 cups
Ingredients:
- 4 cups filtered, preferably alkaline water
- 1 cup of raw almonds
- half teaspoon Himalayan salt or sea salt
- stevia to sweeten if needed

Instructions:
1. First, soak almonds in water with half teaspoon salt (sea salt or Himalayan salt) for about 12 hours.
2. Place in a high-speed blender until the mixture is smooth.
3. Strain using cheesecloth.
4. Place in a blender again, adding some stevia to sweeten if needed.
5. Stir well and place in a fridge.

Asparagus – A Humble Green Superfood

Asparagus is a powerful superfood that is low in calories and high in vitamins, minerals, and antioxidants. It's just perfect for alkaline keto diets and can be added to a variety of foods and dishes, such as soups, salads, vegetable creams, and egg scrambles.

Let's have a look at its amazing benefits...

1. Very Nutritious and Low in Calories

Asparagus is full of vital nutrients. Half cup of asparagus (approximately 100 grams) contains:

Calories: 20
Protein: 2.2 grams
Fat: 0.2 grams
Fiber: 1.8 grams
Vitamin C: 12% of the RDI
Vitamin A: 18% of the RDI
Vitamin K: 57% of the RDI
Folate: 34% of the RDI
Potassium: 6% of the RDI
Phosphorous: 5% of the RDI
Vitamin E: 7% of the RDI
Asparagus also has some traces of iron, zinc, and riboflavin.

Just like watercress, asparagus is very rich in vitamin K, a nutrient you need for optimal blood clotting and bone health.

2. Full of Antioxidants

Asparagus, like other green veggies, contains high levels of antioxidants such as vitamin E, vitamin C, and glutathione.

It's also very rich in the flavonoids: quercetin, isorhamnetin and kaempferol that have been linked to blood pressure-lowering and anti-inflammatory benefits.

3. Great for Your Digestive Health

Asparagus is very rich in insoluble fiber that helps support regular bowel movements. At the same time, it also contains some levels of soluble fiber, which feeds the friendly bacteria in the gut.

4. Excellent Source of Folate

Folate is an important nutrient that helps form red blood cells. It also produces DNA for healthy cell growth. As such, folate is one of the nutrients especially recommended during pre-pregnancy and early pregnancy.

Asparagus

How to Add Asparagus to Your Diet

-add some cooked asparagus to your bacon and eggs
-eat it as a snack with some guacamole or pesto
-cook it and chop it to add it to your salads, omelets and veggie dishes

What I like about asparagus is that it's inexpensive, easy to get, and tasty.

Now, let's try some of my favorite alkaline keto-friendly asparagus recipes.

Asparagus Recipes

Tasty Low Carb Breakfast

Serves:2
Ingredients:
- ¼ lb. pork belly sliced thin or pancetta
- ½ onion diced
- ½ bell pepper diced
- 4 asparagus spears diced
- 1 ½ cups spinach
- 1 tablespoon coconut oil
- ½ teaspoon nutmeg
- 1 teaspoon cumin
- 1 tablespoon diced cilantro
- 1 tablespoon diced parsley
- Pinch of salt
- 2 cups favorite salad greens
- Big squeeze of lemon juice for the salad greens
- 2 eggs

Preparation
1. Put egg and spices in a separate bowl and whisk well, set off to the side.
2. Melt the coconut oil in a frying pan over medium. Fry up the pork. When it is cooked thoroughly and browned, remove and allow to drain on paper towels. Leave the rest of the oil in the pan.
3. Add and sauté the asparagus for three minutes, then add the bell pepper and onion cooking for three more minutes.

Asparagus

4.Mix in the spinach, pork, and egg. Cook for 4-5 minutes until the egg, is set, flipping every so often. Divide into two servings and top with cilantro/parsley. Serve with greens and add a squeeze of lemon.

Veggies in a Cave

Servings - 2 to 3

Ingredients
- 1 onion
- 2 zucchinis
- 8 mushrooms
- 8 asparagus
- 1 leek

Condiments: salt, cumin powder, and olive oil.

Instructions:
1. Wash and chop the vegetables into small or medium-sized pieces.
2. Put on the grill (I use one that does not require using any kind of oil for cooking) set to low heat.
3. Add salt and cumin. Flip occasionally so that your veggies don't burn themselves to death (it takes about 10-15 minutes on low heat).
4. Remove when ready and add a drizzle of olive oil to the plate.
5. Serve and enjoy!

Asparagus

Creamy Asparagus Soup

This soup is easy to prepare and incredibly nourishing!

Serves: 2

Ingredients:

- 1 cup of cooked asparagus
- 1 cup of coconut milk
- A few onion rings
- 1 tablespoon coconut oil
- Half cup water, filtered
- A few lime and lemon slices, peeled
- Himalayan salt and black pepper to taste

Instructions:

1. Blend all the ingredients in a blender until smooth and creamy.
2. Season with more salt and spices if needed.
3. Serve cold or cooked. If needed, add in some protein (hard-boiled eggs, smoked salmon, meat, etc.)
4. Enjoy!

Tomato – The Common-Sense Superfood

Want to have a healthy-looking, glowing skin? Add more tomatoes to your diet. Tomatoes are rich in beta carotene to nourish your skin while protecting it from pre-mature wrinkles and aging.

They are inexpensive, nutritious, and very easy to add to your diet. They always make a delicious and hydrating addition to salads, side dishes, and even smoothies (such as for example, Spanish gazpacho).

Let's have a closer look at all the health benefits of tomato:

1. **It's Very Hydrating and Low in Carbs**

1 middle-sized tomato (approximately 100 grams), contains:

Calories: 18

Water: 95%

Protein: 0.9 grams

Carbs: 3.9 grams

Sugar: 2.6 grams

Fiber: 1.2 grams

Fat: 0.2 grams

Tomato juice can be enjoyed chilled, with some ice cubes, or turned into thick tomato soup or a dip (perfect as a warm and comforting side dish on a cold winter day).

2. Rich in Vitamins and Minerals

Tomatoes are very abundant in Vitamin C (one tomato can provide up to 28% of the recommended daily intake), potassium (good for blood pressure control), Vitamin K1 (essential for bone health and blood clotting), as well as folate (crucial for cell function and tissue growth).

3. Natural Skin Health

Tomatoes are one of the best superfoods for healthy-looking skin. They are very rich in lycopene, a plant compound that may protect your skin against sunburn. At the same time, beta-carotene improves the tone of your skin, making it look more hydrated and glowing.

How to Add More Tomatoes to Your Diet:

-tomatoes taste great in all kinds of salads and side dishes

-they are also an incredibly hydrating snack, simply slice them, add some herbs, Himalayan salt, and olive oil, and enjoy!

-they can be easily blended into dips, creams, and sauces

-they also taste delicious in smoothies and juices

-fresh tomato juice tastes great in green smoothies

Healthy Alkaline Keto Recipes with Tomatoes

The Healthy Skin Glow Bowl

This bowl is designed to help you have a glowing, healthy-looking skin. All this while helping your body get back to balance through optimal nutrition.

Serves 1-2
Ingredients for the Smoothie:
- 1 tablespoon coconut oil
- 1 cup of cashew or other nut milk of your choice
- Half cup broccoli, steamed (you can also use steamed zucchini or cauliflower)
- 1 big tomato
- 1 small garlic clove, peeled
- A handful of fresh cilantro leaves, washed
- Himalayan salt to taste

Ingredients for the Toppings:
- A handful of cashews
- A few avocado slices
- A few cucumber slices

Instructions:
1. Blend all the smoothie ingredients until smooth.
2. Pour into a bowl and add in the toppings.
3. Serve and enjoy!

Tomato

Tomato Alfalfa Soup

Serves: 2

Ingredients:

- 1 large bunch alfalfa leaves
- 2 stems of celery
- ½ red onion
- 1 tsp Himalayan salt
- 1 cup of chopped tomatoes
- ½ cup of boiled water

Instructions:

1. Place all of the ingredients into a blender and process until smooth.

2. Serve at room temperature with a good quality extra-virgin olive oil drizzled over the top, and some alfalfa sprouts if you want.

Tomato

Fresh Tomato Gazpacho

This is a great summer-entertaining dish to add to a meal.

Serves: 4

Ingredients:

- 1 red onion, chopped
- 2 garlic cloves, crushed
- 1 red bell pepper, de-seeded and chopped
- 4-5 ripe tomatoes
- 1 cup of vegetable stock
- 1 ½ cups of sieved tomatoes
- 2 tbsp olive oil
- 1 tsp Himalayan salt
- 3 tbsp Red Wine Vinegar
- Handful of mint leaves

Instructions:

1. Place all of the ingredients into a blender and process until smooth.

2. Place in the fridge overnight to allow the flavors to develop and enjoy cold with extra fresh mint leaves and a drizzle of oil.

Tomato Cilantro Relish

This recipe is perfect for adding as a side to a more substantial, spicy meal or use as a snack with low carb crackers or veggies.

Ingredients:

- 1 large bunch of cilantro, chopped
- 2 tablespoons of chopped mint leaves
- 2 onions, finely chopped
- 1 diced jalapeño pepper
- 1 cup of baby tomatoes, chopped
- 1 lime, zest only

Instructions:

Mix the relish ingredients together and leave to one side. This is better to sit in the fridge for a few hours to allow the flavors to develop. This could be done up to 24 hours in advance.

Celery – The Simple Everyday Superfood

Celery is a Simple Superfood...
Most people think that healthy superfoods are expensive, hard to pronounce, hard to find, and unheard of.

Well, it doesn't have to be that way. There are many simple, common-sense superfoods that are easy to find (in your local grocery store) and can help you take your health to the next level. Celery is one of them, so let's have a look at its primary health and wellness benefits.

The Benefits of Celery
Celery is very rich in:
-vitamin K (an essential vitamin that is needed by the body for blood clotting)
-vitamin A (healthy immune system, anti-age, and good vision)
-vitamins B2 and B6 (better nutrient absorption)
-vitamin C (healthy immune system and sustainable all-day energy)

It is also rich in:
-folate (to make red and white blood cells in the bone marrow, while converting carbohydrates into energy)
-potassium (a mineral and an electrolyte to help your muscles work, as well as nourish the muscles that control your heartbeat and breathing)
-manganese (needed for healthy bones)
-pantothenic acid (to synthesize and metabolize proteins, carbohydrates, and fats)
-dietary fiber (digestive health and regular bowel movements)

Celery

Celery is also very low in calories and sugar, making it a perfect choice for a quick and healthy snack (I love snacking on celery sticks with some hummus or guacamole).

It's an excellent juicing ingredient. When juicing, you give your digestive system a rest, and the nutrients absorb much quicker (and easier) because there is no fiber.

However, if you don't have a juicer, you can also add some celery leaves to your green smoothies.

Recipes with Celery

Celery Juice for Energy & Weight Loss

Avocado oil offers good fat to help you absorb the minerals and vitamins from the juice. I love this juice whenever I need "an injection of energy." Himalayan salt adds alkaline minerals and makes this juice taste amazing. If you like spicy juices, feel free to add in some hot sauce or chili powder.

Servings: 2
Ingredients:
- 1 lemon, peeled
- 1 lime, peeled
- 6 celery stalks, chopped
- A handful of arugula leaves
- 2 big cucumbers, peeled and chopped
- 2 tablespoons avocado oil
- Himalayan salt to taste
- Optional: hot habanero sauce or chili powder

Instructions:
1. Place through a juicer.
2. Juice and combine with the avocado oil and Himalayan salt.
3. Serve in a glass and enjoy!

Celery

On the Go Celery Juice Shot (Liver Lover)

This simple recipe helps detoxify the liver, and it works really well first thing in the morning.

Serves: 1
Ingredients:
- 1 grapefruit, peeled
- Half cup celery leaves
- 1 tablespoon avocado oil or coconut oil
- Half cup of coconut milk
- Stevia to sweeten, if needed

Instructions:
1. Juice grapefruit and celery.
2. In a small glass, combine the juice with the rest of the ingredients.
3. Stir well, drink, and enjoy!
4. To your health!

Celery

Easy Energy Reboot Juice

This recipe uses coconut water to help you spice up your celery juice and make it taste amazing.

Serves: 1-2
Ingredients:
- 1 cup of coconut water
- 1 cup celery leaves
- 1-inch ginger
- 1 grapefruit, peeled
- Ice cubes

Instructions:
1. Juice the celery, ginger, and grapefruit.
2. Combine with coconut water and ice cubes.
3. Serve and enjoy!

Celery

Crazy Keto No Sugar Smoothie

This vegetable, keto-friendly green smoothie is rich in good fats and nutrients. A few spices make it taste delicious!

Servings: 1-2
Ingredients
Liquid:
- 1 cup coconut milk, thick, full-fat
- Half cup almond milk, unsweetened
- 1 tablespoon olive oil
- 1 tablespoon avocado oil

Dry:
- 2 cucumbers, peeled
- 1 big garlic clove, peeled
- 2 small celery sticks
- A handful of green olives, pitted

Other:
- A pinch of Himalaya salt to taste
- Half teaspoon oregano
- A pinch of black pepper to taste

Instructions:
1. Combine all the ingredients in a blender.
2. Process well until smooth.
3. Serve and enjoy!

Celery

Cucumber Kale Alkaline Keto Smoothie

Celery stalks are full of vitamins and minerals, including vitamin K, vitamin A, potassium, and folate. They blend very well with cucumber and creamy nut kinds of milk. All you need to make a super green and tasty smoothie!

Servings: 2
Ingredients
Liquid:
- 1 cup cashew milk
- 1 cup water, filtered, preferably alkaline
- 2 tablespoons lemon juice
- 2 tablespoons avocado oil

Dry:
- 4 celery stalks, chopped
- 2 big cucumbers, peeled and chopped
- 2 tablespoons of cashews

Other:
- Himalayan salt and black pepper to taste
- A pinch of chili or curry powder (optional)

Instructions:
1. Place all the ingredients in a blender.
2. Process well until smooth.
3. Serve and enjoy!

Fennel – The Bulb of Vitality

Perhaps you have tried fennel tea or fennel essential oil. But, have you ever tried eating or juicing a fennel bulb? If not, the time is now!

Fennel bulbs have a mild, licorice-like sweet flavor. They are known for their multiple culinary, antioxidant, and anti-inflammatory properties.

So, let's have a closer look at why fennel bulbs are good for you.

1. Very Nutritious

Fennel bulb is low in calories and high in nutrients. It's particularly rich in vitamin C, a water-soluble vitamin your body needs for immune health, tissue repair, as well as collagen synthesis.

Another important nutrient that fennel bulbs contain is manganese. It is crucial for enzyme activation, an efficient metabolism, blood sugar regulation, and bone development.

Other nutrients found in fennel include potassium, magnesium, and calcium.

2. Rich in Antioxidants

Polyphenol antioxidants found in fennel can lower the risk of many diseases such as: obesity, neurological disorders, and type 2 diabetes.

3. Naturally Sweet

Adding a few slices of fennel bulb to your smoothies and juices will make them tasty, naturally sweet, and delicious.

4. Other Benefits

Fennel may also have antibacterial properties and act as a natural anti-inflammatory.

Fennel

How to Add More Fennel to Your Diet

1. Juice it and use it to flavor your water. Tastes delicious!

2. Blend a few slices into a smoothie. This is perfect for sweet smoothies.

3. Add it to your soups, stews, and salads.

4. Juice it with some greens and a couple of carrots.

Now, let's have a look at the recipes….

Fennel

Energy Fennel Juice

This juice will help you start your day with an abundance of energy. Nothing feels better than knowing you are feeding your body with nutrients first thing in the morning.

Servings: 1-2

Ingredients:

- 1 cup baby spinach
- 2 small carrots, peeled (unless organic)
- Half inch ginger, peeled
- 1 red bell pepper
- Half fennel bulb
- 1 lemon, peeled
- 1 tablespoon avocado oil
- Pinch of Himalayan salt

Instructions:

1. Wash and chop the greens, carrots, fennel, lemon, and bell pepper.

2. Place through a juicer.

3. Pour the juice into a big glass or another utensil of your choice and stir in 1 tablespoon of avocado oil.

4. Add a bit of Himalayan salt to taste.

5. Enjoy and drink to your health!

Fennel

Sweet Balance Juice

Servings: 2
Ingredients:
- 4 big cucumbers, peeled
- Half fennel bulb
- 1-inch ginger, peeled
- 1 big grapefruit, peeled
- 1 lemon, peeled
- Half cup water, filtered

Instructions:
1. Wash and chop all the ingredients.
2. Place through a juicer.
3. Add some water if needed
4. Stir well, drink, and enjoy!

Fennel

Fennel Salad Dressing

Ingredients:
- A few slices of fennel bulb
- ¼ cup avocado oil
- 2 lime slices
- 1 teaspoon Himalayan salt
- 2 tablespoons lemon juice, fresh
- 1 chili flake if you like it spicy

Instructions:
1. Blend all the ingredients.
2. Use as a salad dressing or as a dip to enjoy with raw veggies.

Fennel Detox Soup

Serves: 2

Ingredients:
- Half fennel bulb
- 1 red bell pepper
- 1 cup of coconut milk
- 1 tablespoon coconut oil
- A pinch of nutmeg

Instructions:

Blend and enjoy raw or lightly cooked.

Grapefruit –Why Is It Healthier Than Orange?

I have nothing against oranges, I eat them in moderation and use them in some of my recipes occasionally. They are a very popular fruit where I am originally from, and so is the fruit juice. But here's one thing to understand – oranges are high in sugar. Yes, they also provide Vitamin C and other nutrients. Unfortunately, sugar is still sugar.

In terms of alkaline-acid balance, and foods, oranges are considered acid-forming to the body. This is not because of their acidic taste, but because of their high sugar content. Sugar (natural, processed, fructose, and all kinds of sugar) are very acid-forming to the body.

This is why I am a big fan of grapefruits. They are also very rich in Vitamin C, just like oranges, however, they are low in sugar, and just like limes and lemons, they are considered alkaline-forming fruits.

Low sugar and high alkaline mineral profile is what matters. So, even though acidic in taste (and also a bit bitter), grapefruits are one of the most alkaline-forming foods you could ingest.

And, since they are also very low in sugar, they are totally keto-approved. So, let's have a closer look at all the health and wellness benefits of grapefruits.

Health Benefits of Grapefruit

1. Super Low in Calories, and Very High in Nutrients

The nutritional value of grapefruits speaks for itself:

Only half of a medium-sized grapefruit provides the following:

Calories: 52

Carbs: 13 grams

Protein: 1 gram

Fiber: 2 grams

Vitamin C: 64% of the RDI

Vitamin A: 28% of the RDI

Potassium: 5% of the RDI

Thiamine: 4% of the RDI

Folate: 4% of the RDI

Magnesium: 3% of the RDI

2. Great for Your Immune System

Since grapefruit is high in vitamin C, it can protect your cells from harmful bacteria and viruses. Aside from that, Vitamin C can help you recover or heal your body faster.

Grapefruits are also rich in other minerals and vitamins such as Vitamin A, and these are also crucial for a healthy immune system.

3. Great for Appetite Control and Reduced Sugar Cravings

Grapefruit contains natural fiber, which will help you stay full and control your appetite.

4. Great for Natural Weight Loss

Grapefruit is a very weight loss friendly food because it's high in nutrients and low in calories.

5. Good for Low Sugar and Diabetic Diets

Eating grapefruits may have the potential to prevent insulin resistance. It's just perfect for low sugar and low carb diets.

6. Rich in Antioxidants

Natural antioxidants present in grapefruits (such as Vitamin C and Beta-carotene) help protect your cells from damage caused by free radicals. They also help you get rid of toxins, promoting energy and vitality.

7. Super Hydrating and Full of Alkaline Minerals

Grapefruit contains a lot of water and can be easily juiced. So, if you are sick and tired of drinking "normal water," try some fresh grapefruit juice instead!

Grapefruit

Here are some ways to enjoy grapefruit:

-Peel it and snack on its slices

-Blend it with some coconut cream and stevia to enjoy a naturally sweet, low carb dessert

-Add a few slices to your salads, or add 1-2 tablespoons of its fresh juice to your salad dressings

-Blend it to make a smoothie or add to your favorite low carb smoothies (grapefruits blend very well with coconut milk, almond milk, red bell peppers, avocados, and greens).

Now, let's have a look at some grapefruit recipes!

Grapefruit

Hormone Rebalancer Natural Energy Smoothie

This smoothie recipe is a fantastic option if you don't like green smoothies, but you still want to experience all the health benefits of alkaline keto smoothies.

This recipe uses stevia, which is a natural sweetener, very often used both on keto and alkaline diets.

Although, let me remind you that once your taste buds have adapted, you will be able to do without any sweeteners easily.

Still, if you need one- go for stevia.

Servings: 1-2

Ingredients:

- 1 big grapefruit, peeled and halved
- 1 cup water (filtered, preferably alkaline)
- 1 inch of ginger, peeled
- 1 tablespoon of coconut oil
- Half teaspoon maca powder
- Stevia to sweeten, if desired

Instructions:

1. Blend all the ingredients in a blender.
2. Serve and enjoy!

Grapefruit

Grapefruit Fat Burner Smoothie

This recipe combines the best fat-burning ingredients ever, helps you concentrate for long hours while feeling lighter.

It's also great if you suffer from water retention. I love drinking this smoothie in the summer.

Servings: 2

Ingredients:

- 1 green tea teabag (or 1 teaspoon green tea powder)
- 1 horsetail infusion tea bag (or 1 teaspoon horsetail infusion powder)
- 1 cup of water, filtered
- 1 big avocado, peeled and pitted
- 1 big grapefruit
- Half cup of coconut milk
- 1 teaspoon cinnamon powder
- Stevia to sweeten

Instructions:
1. Boil 1 cup of water.
2. Add in the green tea and horsetail infusion.
3. Cover.
4. In the meantime, process the remaining ingredients in a blender.
5. Add in the cooled herbal infusion and process again.
6. If needed sweeten with stevia. Serve and enjoy!

Grapefruit

Delicious Vitamin C Power House

This recipe is full of Vitamin C to help you strengthen your immune system and feel amazing! It also sneaks in some greens to make it even healthier!

Serves: 1-2
Ingredients for the Smoothie:
- Half cup of blueberries or raspberries (fresh or frozen)
- 1 grapefruit, peeled
- Half cup of baby spinach leaves
- A few fresh mint leaves
- Optional: stevia to sweeten

Ingredients for the Toppings:
- A handful of crushed almonds
- 1 tablespoon chia seeds
- 2 slices of apple

Instructions
1. Blend all the smoothie ingredients until smooth. If you are making this smoothie on a hot summer day, feel free to add some ice cubes. Pour the smoothie into a bowl.
2. Mix in the rest of the ingredients by adding them on top.
3. You can enjoy your smoothie bowl now or store it in the fridge for later.

Grapefruit Weight Loss Tonic

This quick tonic recipe is perfect for hot summers and will help you stay energized for hours.

Serves: 1-2
Ingredients:
- 2 big grapefruits
- 1-inch ginger, peeled
- 1 tablespoon avocado oil
- A few ice cubes
- 1 cup of water
- Green tea or black tea

Instructions:
1. Boil the water and make your tea (use 1 teabag per 1 cup of water).
2. Leave covered and let it cool down.
3. In the meantime, juice the grapefruits and ginger.
4. Now combine the tea with ice cubes and add in the juice.
5. Stir in the avocado oil, mix well, and, if needed, add more ice cubes.
6. Enjoy!

****If you don't have a juicer, just blend all the ingredients in a blender: 1 cup of tea (cooled down), grapefruits, ginger, and avocado oil. Add some water if needed.

Coconut Oil Magic – The All In One Solution?

Coconut oil is probably the most famous oil out there. It has been called a superfood and miracle oil many times. And, as a Celebrity Oil, it surely lives up to its expectations!

Its unique combination of fatty acids has many health benefits such as boosting fat loss, improving heart health, and brain function.

Coconut oil has numerous wellness powers, such as:

1. Healthy fatty acids

Coconut oil is very rich in certain saturated fats that have very positive effects on the body:

-They can stimulate fat burn while providing a quick energy boost. -They raise HDL (good) cholesterol in your blood (some studies say that HDL may help reduce heart disease risk.)

So, what is the difference between most dietary fats and coconut oil?

Most dietary fats are categorized as long-chain triglycerides (LCTs). Coconut oil, on the other hand, contains some medium-chain triglycerides (MCTs), which are shorter fatty acid chains.

When you eat medium-chain triglycerides (MCTs), they go straight to your liver. Then, your body can automatically use them as a quick source of energy (it can also turn them into ketones).

Ketones are especially beneficial for your brain. Many studies point to ketones as a possible treatment for epilepsy, Alzheimer's disease, and other medical conditions.

2. Improved heart health

Coconut oil is one of the most popular health foods in the Western World. But, it's still relatively new in our culture, and we surely haven't been consuming it for hundreds of years. The question is – what could be the long-term benefits of using coconut oil regularly?

Well, a fascinating fact is that some countries have been using coconut oil as one of the main "staple foods" in their diets. Many people living in those countries have been using coconut oil for generations. An example of that are the people of a small island chain in the South Pacific, called Tokelau. Most of them obtained about 60% of their calories from coconuts and coconut oil. The heart disease rate in Tokealu was extremely low, and most people enjoyed excellent health.

Was it because of the coconut only? Could other factors and lifestyle choices influence that as well? Perhaps, it's their genetics?

Well, it's up to you to make your decision. For me, it's one of the examples of how coconut oil can positively influence our health if we choose to use it.

Another example, similar to the Tokelau islands, are Kitavan people in Papua, New Guinea. They also eat a lot of coconuts (as well as fresh fruit and fish) and hardly ever suffer from heart disease. Once again, this could also be due to the climate, genetics, and other foods they consume as well as their overall healthy, natural, and real food lifestyle. However, the one thing they have in common is that they have been consuming coconut and coconut oil for generations.

3. A fat that burns fat?

I talk to my readers and newsletter subscribers regularly. They all have different health goals they wish to reach. However, the number one health goal that most of the people I talk to wish to accomplish is weight loss and fat burn. And even those who have already reached their weight loss goals, still continue their "healthy weight loss" journey because they want to maintain the results of their effort and hard work.

Some people think weight loss or weight gain is just a matter of how many calories we eat. While there is some truth to that calories in and out theory (and it makes sense), the source of the calories is very important too. You see, different foods affect your body and your hormones in different ways. For example, you could eat 2000 processed calories from an unhealthy fast-food meal that satisfies your dopamine levels for a short period of time (while leaving your body malnourished and hungry, not to mention the damage caused by all the chemicals, processed sugars, and carbs from fast food). Or, you could eat 2000 calories from a healthy, clean food source to feed and nourish your body and create balance so that you no longer crave processed sugars, and weight loss becomes easier.

You see, the already mentioned, miraculous MCTs in coconut oil can speed up the number of calories your body burns compared with longer-chain fatty acids.

Aside from that, coconut oil is clean, healthy, and natural food. As such, it offers quality, unprocessed calories.

Word of caution, though. Some people treat coconut oil as a health and weight loss shortcut. What I mean by that is an exaggeration. You hear some food is good for you and so you overdo it to get the results fast. Well, common-sense should be your best friend! Coconut oil, by itself, will not work wonders on your health and life. It's all about changing your lifestyle, eating a clean food diet, and moving your body. Then, use coconut oil as a natural supplement, for example, have a tablespoon of coconut oil when craving sugar or processed sweets. Or add some to your smoothies.

Also remember, even the healthiest superfood can harm you if you overdo it or try to use it as a shortcut. And yes, it is high in calories.

So, for some people, it can lead to weight gain if eaten in large amounts (and from a place of "I don't want to change my diet and lifestyle, I just want some new superfood to work wonders for me").

We will come back to weight loss with coconut oil later in the recipe section. However, if weight loss is your goal, I highly recommend you read my book: *Alkaline Ketogenic Lifestyle for Massive Weight Loss* (Alkaline Keto Diet book #6) which you can order from Amazon (Kindle and paperback, audio coming soon). It's a short read, but it's very to the point. It will help you determine what to focus on to lose weight and keep it off, without sacrificing your health, hormone balance, and sanity.

So now, let's have a look at different kinds of coconut oil so that you know which one to buy.

Unrefined Organic Coconut Oil

This type of oil offers the best of the benefits listed above. It is extracted from fresh coconut. Since only a wet-milled fermentation process is used, the beneficial properties of the coconut remain untouched. This exact type of coconut oil has been proven to have the highest antioxidant levels. Even though this process does use heat, the studies show that it does not harm the oil or reduce nutrient levels.

"Extra Virgin" Coconut Oil

"Extra Virgin" is an excellent standard for olive oil but not for coconut oil. This is produced by cold-pressing the oil, and this process does not preserve the antioxidants as well.

Refined Coconut Oils

Refined coconut oil is usually tasteless and has no coconut smell. It is very often heated, bleached, and deodorized. Even though healthy options are available, many refined coconut oils do not have the benefits of unrefined.

Fractionated Oil or MCT Oil

Fractionated oil or MCT oil is liquid coconut oil. What makes it different from unrefined oils is that it does not get solid below 76 degrees. Unfortunately, it doesn't contain all of the beneficial properties of unrefined coconut oil.

What Type of Coconut Oil to Use?

For external uses (hair or skincare) expeller-pressed, fractionated, or other types of refined coconut oil are fine, but for internal use, unrefined organic oil is best.

Now, let's have a look at some amazing coconut oil recipes!

Coconut Oil Recipes

Green Dream Weight Loss Smoothie

This green vegetable smoothie blends the best of the alkaline and keto worlds. It's my number one recommendation if your goal is weight loss. It may take some time to get used to green vegetable smoothies. Especially if you are more accustomed to drinking "sweety-carby-fruity" smoothies (not that good for you, unfortunately).

But trust me, after a few green smoothies, and fantastic energy they provide, you will be wondering how you could ever live without them.

Servings: 2

Ingredients:

- 1 cup coconut or almond milk (unsweetened)
- 1 cup water (filtered, preferably alkaline)
- 1 small avocado, peeled and pitted
- A handful of spinach
- 2 tablespoons of coconut oil
- Pinch of Himalaya salt to taste

Instructions:

1. Place all the ingredients in a blender.
2. Blend well.
3. Serve and enjoy!

Immune System Energy Smoothie

This is a super simple alkaline green smoothie that will help you boost your immune system by enriching your diet with vitamin C and a myriad of alkaline minerals.

Serves 1-2

Ingredients

- 2 big limes, peeled
- 1 cup of coconut or almond milk
- A handful of kale leaves, washed
- Optional- a few drops of liquid chlorophyll
- 1 lime wedge to garnish (1 per serving)
- 1-2 tablespoons coconut oil
- 1 teaspoon cinnamon powder
- Stevia to sweeten, if needed

Instructions

1. Place in a blender.
2. Process until smooth.
3. Serve in a smoothie glass and garnish with a wedge of lime.
4. Enjoy!

Coconut Oil

Coconut Oil Cortado Style Coffee Recipe

This recipe is perfect if you are not a breakfast person!

Ingredients:
- 1 expresso
- 1 tablespoon coconut oil
- 2-4 tablespoons coconut milk

Instructions:
1. Combine all the ingredients in a small coffee cup.
2. Mix well, drink, and enjoy!

Creamy Cinnamon Latte Recipe

Cinnamon makes this coffee taste so nice, and it also prevents sugar cravings- we always want to tackle the problem from different angles!

Ingredients:
- 1 cup coconut milk, warm
- 1 expresso
- 2 tablespoons coconut oil
- 1 teaspoon cinnamon

Stevia to sweeten, if needed.

Instructions:
1. Blend all the ingredients in a hand blender.
2. Shake well, serve, and enjoy!

Green Tea Weight Loss Drink

This simple tea-based drink is perfect as a quick afternoon pick me up!

Ingredients:
- 1 cup of green tea
- 1 cup of coconut milk
- 2 tablespoons coconut oil
- Stevia to sweeten if needed

Instructions:
Blend all the ingredients, serve, and enjoy!

Easy Creamy Warm Salmon Salad

Salmon is one of my favorite keto ingredients, especially to use for quick, nourishing salads like this one.

Servings: 1-2

Ingredients:

- Half cup raw cashews, crushed
- 4 slices of smoked salmon
- 2 tablespoons of coconut oil
- 1 cup fresh spinach
- 2 tomatoes, sliced
- Himalayan salt and black pepper to taste
- A few thin slices of cheddar cheese

Instructions:

1. Place coconut oil in a frying pan.
2. Switch on the heat (medium heat).
3. Add the spinach and Himalaya salt and stir-fry until soft.
4. Now, add the salmon, cashews, and tomato slices.
5. Stir fry until the salmon is warm.
6. Take off the heat and place in a salad bowl.
7. If needed, add more Himalayan salt to taste.
8. Top up with some cheddar cheese, serve and enjoy!

Ridiculously Easy Sweet Alkaline Keto Balls

This recipe is a must-try to help you:

-satisfy your "sweet tooth" without eating crappy carbs or sugars

-add in some good fats and anti-inflammatory properties too

-sneak in some alkaline keto superfoods to make sure you stay energized

Ingredients:

- 1 cup raw cashews (unsalted, unsweetened), soaked for at least 4 hours
- 1 cup raw almonds (unsalted, unsweetened), soaked for at least 4 hours
- 4 tablespoons coconut oil
- 4 tablespoons coconut milk
- 1 tablespoon cinnamon powder

Instructions:

1. Place all the ingredients in a high-speed blender or a food processor.
2. Using your hands, form the "dough" into small balls.
3. Place the balls on a big plate and put them in a fridge for a few hours.
4. Serve and enjoy!

More Alkaline Keto Books

Join Our VIP Readers' Newsletter to Boost Your Wellbeing

Would you like to be notified about our new health and wellness books? How about receiving them at deeply discounted prices?

What about awesome giveaways, latest health tips, and motivation?

If that is something you are interested in, please visit the link below to join our newsletter:

www.yourwellnessbooks.com/email-newsletter

As a bonus, you will receive a free complimentary eBook *Alkaline Paleo Superfoods*

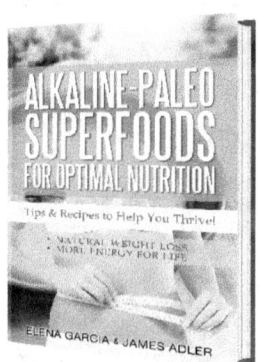

Sign up link:

www.yourwellnessbooks.com/email-newsletter

(any technical problems with your sign up, please email: info@yourwellnessbooks.com)

More Books & Resources in the Healthy Lifestyle Series
Available at:

www.yourwellnessbooks.com

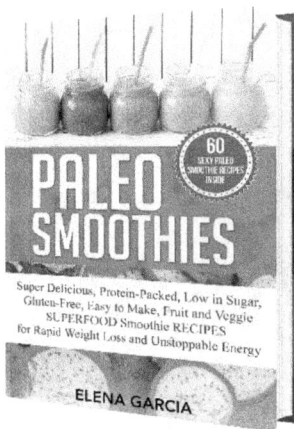
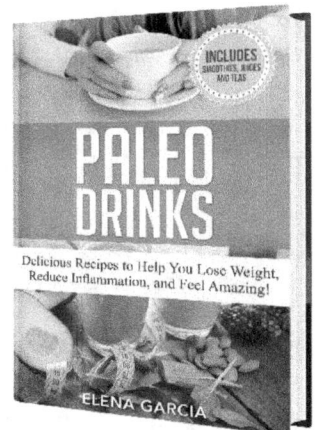
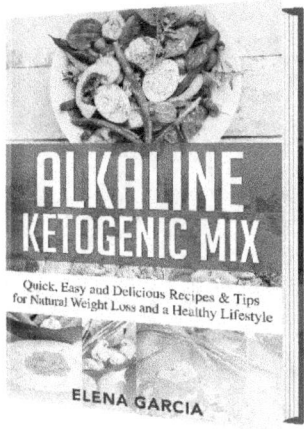
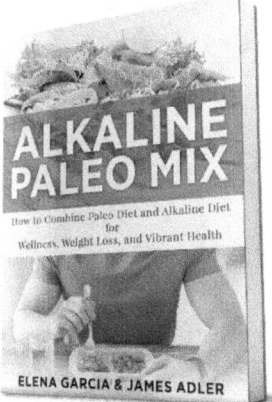

More Alkaline Keto Books

Until next time, wishing you all the best on your journey!

Elena & Your Wellness Books Team

www.YourWellnessBooks.com

We Need Your Help

One more thing, before you go, could you please do us a quick favor?

It would be great if you could leave us a short review on Amazon.

Don't worry, it doesn't have to be long. One sentence is enough.

Let others know your favorite recipes and who you think this book can help.

Your review can inspire more and more people to turn to the alkaline ketogenic lifestyle so that they can finally achieve their wellness and weight loss goals the way they deserve.

Your honest review is critical.

Thank You for your support!

More Alkaline Keto Books

www.ingramcontent.com/pod-product-compliance
Lightning Source LLC
Chambersburg PA
CBHW071355080526
44587CB00017B/3115